CARDIOLOGY PEARLS

Key Insights for Clinical Practice

Dr Essam Abdelhakim

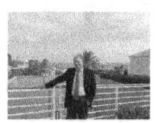

Copyright © 2024 Dr Essam Abdelhakim

All rights reserved

The characters and events portrayed in this book are fictitious. Any similarity to real persons, living or dead, is coincidental and not intended by the author.

No part of this book may be reproduced, or stored in a retrieval system, or transmitted in any form or by any means, electronic, mechanical, photocopying, recording, or otherwise, without express written permission of the publisher.

Cover design by: Art Painter
Library of Congress Control Number: 2018675309
Printed in the United States of America

CONTENTS

Title Page
Copyright
Introduction
Disclosure

Chapter 1: Introduction to Cardiology	1
Chapter 2: Ischemic Heart Disease (IHD)	6
Chapter 3: Heart Failure	12
Chapter 4: Valvular Heart Diseases	18
Chapter 5: Arrhythmias	24
Chapter 6: Hypertension	30
Chapter 7: Congenital Heart Diseases (Adults)	35
Chapter 8: Cardiomyopathies	42
Chapter 9: Infective Endocarditis and Rheumatic Heart Disease	51
Chapter 11: Cardiac Imaging and Diagnostics	59
Chapter 12: Preventive Cardiology	64
Chapter 13: Cardiology Emergencies	71
Chapter 14: Special Populations in Cardiology	76
About The Author	85

INTRODUCTION

Cardiology Pearls is designed as a practical guide for medical professionals, from residents to experienced cardiologists, looking to sharpen their knowledge and enhance their clinical skills.

This book takes a case-based approach, offering pearls of wisdom that combine evidence-based practices with clinical insights to provide actionable knowledge. Each chapter delves into key areas of cardiology, from ischemic heart disease and heart failure to arrhythmias and congenital heart defects, offering high-yield information that is relevant for day-to-day clinical practice.

Target Audience

- **Medical students** looking to deepen their understanding of cardiology and prepare for clinical exams.
- **Residents** in internal medicine, cardiology, and emergency medicine seeking high-yield clinical scenarios and management pearls.
- **General practitioners** and **primary care physicians** who need to identify and manage common and urgent cardiovascular conditions.
- **Cardiologists** and specialists in the field who want to refresh their knowledge or incorporate the latest treatment strategies into their practice.

DISCLOSURE

Disclosure

This book has been created with the assistance of *Artificial Intelligence (AI) tools* and thoroughly reviewed and edited by the author to ensure clarity, relevance, and educational value.

While every effort has been made to provide accurate and up-to-date information, this content is intended solely for educational and informational purposes.

The author is a medical professional; however, the information provided in this book *is not a substitute for professional medical advice, diagnosis, or treatment.*

Readers are strongly advised to consult licensed healthcare providers or specialists for any medical concerns or conditions.

By using this book, **you acknowledge and agree** that the author shall not be held responsible or liable for any loss, damage, or harm whether physical, emotional, financial, or otherwise that may occur *as a result of the use or misuse of the information presented herein.*

CHAPTER 1: INTRODUCTION TO CARDIOLOGY

Anatomy and Physiology of the Heart
The heart is a muscular organ that serves as the pump of the circulatory system, ensuring oxygenated blood is delivered to the body and deoxygenated blood is sent to the lungs.

Key Pearls On Anatomy And Physiology

1. **Chambers of the Heart:**
    - **Right Atrium (RA):** Receives deoxygenated blood from the superior and inferior vena cava.
    - **Right Ventricle (RV):** Pumps blood into the pulmonary artery for oxygenation.
    - **Left Atrium (LA):** Receives oxygenated blood from the pulmonary veins.
    - **Left Ventricle (LV):** Pumps oxygenated blood into the aorta; the most muscular chamber due to the high-pressure systemic circulation.

    Clinical Pearl:
    - Left ventricular hypertrophy (LVH) is often a marker of chronic hypertension and can predispose to heart failure and arrhythmias.

2. **Heart Valves:**
    - **Atrioventricular (AV) Valves:**

- Tricuspid valve (RA → RV)
- Mitral valve (LA → LV)
- **Semilunar Valves**:
  - Pulmonary valve (RV → pulmonary artery)
  - Aortic valve (LV → aorta)

Clinical Pearl:
- Systolic murmurs over the aortic area often indicate aortic stenosis, especially in elderly patients with a history of calcification.

3. **Coronary Arteries**:
   - Right Coronary Artery (RCA): Supplies the right heart, inferior wall of the LV, and AV node.
   - Left Main Coronary Artery (LMCA): Divides into:
     - Left Anterior Descending (LAD): Supplies the anterior wall of the LV and interventricular septum.
     - Left Circumflex (LCx): Supplies the lateral wall of the LV.

Clinical Pearl:
- LAD occlusion, often termed the "widowmaker," is associated with high mortality if not promptly treated.

4. **Electrical System of the Heart**:
   - **Sinoatrial (SA) Node**: The natural pacemaker of the heart.
   - **Atrioventricular (AV) Node**: Slows conduction, allowing ventricular filling.
   - **Bundle of His and Purkinje Fibers**: Conduct impulses to the ventricles for coordinated

contraction.

Clinical Pearl:
- A prolonged PR interval (>200 ms) on ECG indicates first-degree AV block, often seen in older adults or with beta-blocker use.

Overview of Common Cardiac Conditions

1. **Ischemic Heart Disease (IHD):**
   - Caused by atherosclerosis of coronary arteries, leading to reduced blood flow to the myocardium.
   - Includes **stable angina**, **unstable angina**, **NSTEMI**, and **STEMI**.

Clinical Pearl:
- Nitroglycerin relieves chest pain in angina but not in myocardial infarction; persistence of pain after administration warrants urgent intervention.

2. **Heart Failure (HF):**
   - The heart's inability to pump effectively, leading to fluid overload and poor perfusion.
   - Divided into:
     - HFrEF (reduced ejection fraction, ≤40%).
     - HFpEF (preserved ejection fraction, >50%).

Clinical Pearl:
- BNP and NT-proBNP levels are essential biomarkers for diagnosing and managing heart failure exacerbations.

3. **Arrhythmias:**

- Includes atrial fibrillation, ventricular tachycardia, and bradyarrhythmias.
- Atrial fibrillation is the most common sustained arrhythmia, increasing stroke risk.

Clinical Pearl:
- CHADS2 and CHA2DS2-VASc scores guide anticoagulation therapy in atrial fibrillation patients.

4. **Valvular Heart Disease**:
   - Common causes include calcification (aortic stenosis), rheumatic fever (mitral stenosis), and endocarditis.

Clinical Pearl:
- Listen for murmurs: Diastolic murmurs are always pathological and require further investigation.

5. **Hypertension**:
   - A leading risk factor for ischemic heart disease, heart failure, and stroke.
   - Often asymptomatic until complications occur.

Clinical Pearl:
- Early intervention with lifestyle changes and antihypertensives can prevent target organ damage.

6. **Congenital Heart Diseases**:
   - Persisting into adulthood in many cases, such as atrial septal defects or Tetralogy of

Fallot.

Clinical Pearl:
- Cyanosis in adults may suggest an undiagnosed congenital shunt, such as Eisenmenger syndrome.

7. **Infective Endocarditis:**
    - Infection of the heart valves or endocardium.
    - Common in patients with prosthetic valves or intravenous drug use.

Clinical Pearl:
- Always suspect infective endocarditis in patients with fever and new-onset murmur.

CHAPTER 2: ISCHEMIC HEART DISEASE (IHD)

Ischemic Heart Disease (IHD) encompasses a spectrum of conditions caused by myocardial ischemia, often due to coronary artery disease (CAD). IHD is a leading cause of morbidity and mortality worldwide.

Acute Coronary Syndromes (Acs)

ACS refers to a spectrum of conditions caused by acute myocardial ischemia and includes:

1. **ST-Elevation Myocardial Infarction (STEMI)**
2. **Non-ST-Elevation Myocardial Infarction (NSTEMI)**
3. **Unstable Angina (UA)**

1. STEMI

STEMI results from complete occlusion of a coronary artery, causing transmural ischemia.

Clinical Presentation:
- Chest pain: Sudden, severe, retrosternal, lasting >20 minutes, not relieved by rest or nitroglycerin.
- May radiate to the jaw, left arm, or back.
- Associated symptoms: Diaphoresis, nausea, dyspnea, and anxiety.

Diagnostic Features:
- ECG: ST-segment elevation in two contiguous leads or new-onset left bundle branch block (LBBB).
- Cardiac enzymes: Elevated troponin and CK-MB.

Management:
- **Primary PCI**: Gold standard; aim for a door-to-balloon time of <90 minutes.
- **Thrombolysis**: For centers without PCI access; within 30 minutes of hospital arrival.

Pearl:
- Always assess for contraindications to thrombolysis (e.g., recent stroke, active bleeding).

2. NSTEMI

NSTEMI is caused by partial occlusion of a coronary artery.

Clinical Presentation:
- Similar to STEMI but less severe.

Diagnostic Features:
- ECG: ST depression, T-wave inversion, or nonspecific changes.
- Cardiac enzymes: Elevated troponin confirms myocardial injury.

Management:
- **Anticoagulation**: Enoxaparin or unfractionated heparin.
- **Early PCI**: Within 24-72 hours in high-risk patients (e.g., TIMI score ≥3).

Pearl:
- Elevated troponins without ECG changes can indicate NSTEMI; rely on serial testing for trends.

3. Unstable Angina (UA)

UA is characterized by myocardial ischemia without myocardial necrosis.

Clinical Presentation:
- New-onset angina, worsening angina, or angina at rest.
- No elevation in cardiac biomarkers.

Management:
- Similar to NSTEMI but without the need for serial troponins.
- Focus on risk stratification and anti-ischemic therapy.

Pearl:
- Always differentiate UA from NSTEMI using serial troponin levels.

Chronic Coronary Syndromes (Ccs)

Chronic coronary syndromes result from stable atherosclerotic plaques limiting blood flow during increased myocardial demand.

1. Stable Angina
- **Pathophysiology**: Demand-supply mismatch due to fixed coronary stenosis.
- **Clinical Presentation**: Predictable chest pain triggered by exertion or emotional stress, relieved by rest or nitroglycerin.

Diagnostic Features:
- ECG: Normal at rest, may show ST depression during exertion.
- Stress testing: Inducible ischemia confirms diagnosis.

Management:

- Anti-anginal medications: Beta-blockers, calcium channel blockers, and nitrates.
- Secondary prevention: Aspirin, statins, and lifestyle modification.

Pearl:
- Always assess functional capacity and symptom burden to guide revascularization decisions.

2. Microvascular Angina

- **Pathophysiology**: Dysfunction of small coronary vessels, common in women and diabetic patients.
- **Clinical Presentation**: Angina-like symptoms but normal coronary angiography.
- **Management**: Focus on symptom control with beta-blockers, ACE inhibitors, and lifestyle changes.

Pearl:
- Coronary microvascular dysfunction should be suspected in patients with typical angina and normal angiograms.

High-Yield Management Strategies

1. Dual Antiplatelet Therapy (DAPT)
- Combination of aspirin and a P2Y12 inhibitor (e.g., clopidogrel, ticagrelor, prasugrel).
- Duration:
  - ACS: 12 months.
  - Stable angina post-PCI: 6 months.

Pearl:
- Avoid prasugrel in patients with a history of stroke or age >75 years.

2. Percutaneous Coronary Intervention (PCI)
- Preferred for STEMI, NSTEMI, and refractory stable angina.
- Drug-eluting stents reduce restenosis risk.

Pearl:
- Always assess for stent thrombosis risk factors: noncompliance with DAPT, diabetes, and small vessel size.

3. Coronary Artery Bypass Grafting (CABG)
- Indications:
  - Left main coronary artery disease.
  - Triple-vessel disease in diabetics.
  - Refractory angina not amenable to PCI.

Pearl:
- CABG offers mortality benefits in diabetics with multivessel disease compared to PCI.

Pearls For Interpreting Stress Tests And Angiograms

1. Stress Tests

- **Exercise ECG**: First-line for low-risk patients.
- **Stress Echo**: Preferred in patients with baseline ECG abnormalities.
- **Nuclear Stress Test or Stress MRI**: High sensitivity for ischemia.

Pearl:

- Positive stress test findings: ST depression ≥1 mm, reduced perfusion on imaging, or wall motion abnormalities.

2. Coronary Angiography

- Gold standard for diagnosing coronary artery disease.
- **Findings**:
    - Significant stenosis: ≥70% in major vessels or ≥50% in the left main.

Pearl:

- Fractional flow reserve (FFR) helps determine the functional significance of borderline lesions.

CHAPTER 3: HEART FAILURE

Heart failure (HF) is a complex syndrome characterized by the heart's inability to pump blood effectively to meet the metabolic demands of the body. It can result from structural or functional cardiac abnormalities and is associated with significant morbidity and mortality.

Types Of Heart Failure

Heart failure is classified based on ejection fraction (EF), which is a measure of the percentage of blood the left ventricle pumps out during each contraction.

1. Heart Failure with Reduced Ejection Fraction (HFrEF)
- **Definition**: EF <40%.
- **Pathophysiology**: Systolic dysfunction due to impaired myocardial contractility.
- **Common Causes**:
    - Ischemic heart disease.
    - Dilated cardiomyopathy.
    - Myocarditis.

Pearl:
- HFrEF is the most extensively studied type of HF, with numerous evidence-based therapies available.

2. Heart Failure with Preserved Ejection Fraction (HFpEF)

- **Definition**: EF ≥50%.
- **Pathophysiology**: Diastolic dysfunction due to impaired myocardial relaxation and increased ventricular stiffness.
- **Common Causes**:
    - Hypertension.
    - Obesity.
    - Atrial fibrillation.

Pearl:
- HFpEF is challenging to treat, with management focusing on controlling comorbidities.

3. Heart Failure with Mid-Range Ejection Fraction (HFmrEF)
- **Definition**: EF 41–49%.
- **Pathophysiology**: Features of both systolic and diastolic dysfunction.
- **Common Causes**: Similar to HFrEF and HFpEF.

Pearl:
- HFmrEF patients may benefit from therapies used for HFrEF, though data are limited.

Common Etiologies Of Heart Failure

1. Ischemic Heart Disease (IHD)
- Most common cause of HFrEF.
- Recurrent myocardial infarctions lead to ventricular remodeling and reduced contractility.

Pearl:

- Always assess for coronary artery disease in newly diagnosed HF patients.

2. Non-Ischemic Causes

- **Hypertension**: Common in HFpEF due to increased afterload.
- **Valvular Heart Disease**: Aortic stenosis and mitral regurgitation are significant contributors.
- **Cardiomyopathies**:
  - Dilated: Alcohol, toxins, or genetic mutations.
  - Hypertrophic: Often genetic.
  - Restrictive: Amyloidosis or sarcoidosis.

Pearl:

- Non-ischemic HF often requires a broader diagnostic workup, including imaging and biopsy in select cases.

Management Strategies

1. Guideline-Directed Medical Therapy (GDMT)

GDMT forms the cornerstone of HF management, particularly for HFrEF.

- **Angiotensin-Converting Enzyme Inhibitors (ACEIs)/ Angiotensin Receptor Blockers (ARBs)**: Reduce mortality and morbidity.
- **Beta-Blockers**: Carvedilol, bisoprolol, and metoprolol succinate are proven to improve survival.
- **Mineralocorticoid Receptor Antagonists (MRAs)**: Eplerenone and spironolactone are beneficial in reducing hospitalizations.
- **Sodium-Glucose Cotransporter 2 (SGLT2) Inhibitors**:

Empagliflozin and dapagliflozin improve outcomes in HFrEF.
- **ARNI (Sacubitril/Valsartan)**: Superior to ACEIs/ARBs in HFrEF.

Pearl:
- Titrate GDMT to the maximum tolerated doses for optimal benefit.

2. Diuretics
- Used to relieve congestion and fluid overload.
- **Loop Diuretics**: Furosemide and torsemide are first-line for volume management.

Pearl:
- Monitor for electrolyte imbalances (e.g., hypokalemia, hypomagnesemia) with loop diuretics.

3. Device Therapy
- **Cardiac Resynchronization Therapy (CRT)**:
  - Indicated for patients with EF ≤35%, left bundle branch block (LBBB), and QRS >150 ms despite optimal medical therapy.
- **Implantable Cardioverter Defibrillator (ICD)**:
  - Reduces sudden cardiac death in patients with EF ≤35% and symptomatic HF.

Pearl:
- Assess QRS morphology and duration to determine CRT candidacy.

Acute Decompensated Heart Failure (Adhf)

ADHF is characterized by a rapid onset of symptoms and signs of HF, often requiring urgent medical attention.

Clinical Features:
- Dyspnea at rest or with minimal exertion.
- Orthopnea and paroxysmal nocturnal dyspnea.
- Peripheral edema, ascites, and jugular venous distension.

Pearl:
- Use BNP or NT-proBNP levels to differentiate between cardiac and non-cardiac causes of dyspnea.

Key Management Tips for ADHF

1. **Initial Stabilization:**
   - Supplemental oxygen for hypoxia.
   - Non-invasive ventilation (e.g., CPAP) in severe pulmonary edema.

2. **Volume Overload Management:**
   - **Intravenous Loop Diuretics**: Start promptly to relieve congestion.
   - Monitor urine output and adjust doses as needed.

3. **Hemodynamic Support:**
   - **Inotropes (e.g., dobutamine)**: For patients with hypotension and evidence of low cardiac output.
   - **Vasodilators (e.g., nitroglycerin)**: To reduce preload and afterload in hypertensive ADHF.

4. **Identify and Treat Underlying Causes:**
   - Myocardial infarction, arrhythmias,

infections, or medication non-compliance.

Pearl:

- Early diuresis and hemodynamic optimization are critical to improving outcomes.

CHAPTER 4: VALVULAR HEART DISEASES

Valvular heart diseases (VHD) encompass a wide spectrum of conditions involving dysfunction of one or more heart valves, leading to stenosis (restricted valve opening) or regurgitation (inadequate closure). These conditions significantly impact hemodynamics, potentially resulting in heart failure, arrhythmias, and other complications.

Aortic Valve Disorders

1. Aortic Stenosis (AS)

- **Pathophysiology**: Narrowing of the aortic valve causes increased afterload, left ventricular hypertrophy, and eventual heart failure.
- **Etiology**:
    - Degenerative calcification (most common in elderly patients).
    - Congenital bicuspid aortic valve.
    - Rheumatic heart disease.
- **Clinical Features**:
    - Symptoms: Exertional dyspnea, angina, syncope.
    - Murmur: Harsh systolic crescendo-decrescendo murmur best heard at the right upper sternal border.
- **Management**:
    - Symptomatic severe AS or EF <50% requires

intervention:
- Surgical aortic valve replacement (SAVR).
- Transcatheter aortic valve replacement (TAVR) for high-risk or inoperable patients.

Pearl:
- Severe AS is characterized by a valve area <1.0 cm², mean gradient ≥40 mmHg, or a peak velocity ≥4 m/s.

2. Aortic Regurgitation (AR)
- **Pathophysiology**: Incompetent valve allows blood to flow back into the left ventricle during diastole, leading to volume overload and left ventricular dilation.
- **Etiology**:
    - Acute: Endocarditis, aortic dissection, trauma.
    - Chronic: Bicuspid aortic valve, rheumatic disease, connective tissue disorders (e.g., Marfan syndrome).
- **Clinical Features**:
    - Symptoms: Dyspnea, fatigue, palpitations, angina in severe cases.
    - Murmur: Diastolic decrescendo murmur best heard at the left sternal border.
- **Management**:
    - Acute AR: Emergent surgery.
    - Chronic AR: Surgery indicated in symptomatic patients or asymptomatic patients with significant left ventricular dysfunction (EF ≤50%).

Pearl:

- Look for peripheral signs in chronic AR (e.g., wide pulse pressure, bounding pulses, Quincke's sign).

Mitral Valve Disorders

1. Mitral Stenosis (MS)
- **Pathophysiology**: Obstruction to left ventricular inflow during diastole leads to increased left atrial pressure and pulmonary congestion.
- **Etiology**:
    - Rheumatic fever (most common).
    - Congenital MS (rare).
- **Clinical Features**:
    - Symptoms: Exertional dyspnea, orthopnea, hemoptysis, atrial fibrillation.
    - Murmur: Low-pitched diastolic rumble with an opening snap, best heard at the apex.
- **Management**:
    - Symptomatic patients: Percutaneous balloon mitral valvuloplasty (preferred if anatomy is suitable).
    - Severe cases: Mitral valve replacement.

Pearl:
- The presence of an opening snap indicates pliable leaflets, favoring valvuloplasty.

2. Mitral Regurgitation (MR)
- **Pathophysiology**: Incompetent mitral valve leads to retrograde blood flow into the left atrium during systole, causing volume overload.
- **Etiology**:
    - Acute: Papillary muscle rupture (e.g., post-

MI), endocarditis, chordae tendineae rupture.
- Chronic: Mitral valve prolapse, rheumatic disease, ischemic heart disease.

- **Clinical Features**:
  - Symptoms: Dyspnea, fatigue, palpitations, heart failure in severe cases.
  - Murmur: Holosystolic murmur best heard at the apex radiating to the axilla.

- **Management**:
  - Acute MR: Emergency surgery.
  - Chronic MR: Surgery indicated in symptomatic patients or asymptomatic patients with left ventricular dysfunction (EF ≤60%).

Pearl:
- Mitral valve repair is preferred over replacement when feasible, as it preserves ventricular function.

Tricuspid And Pulmonary Valve Disorders

1. Tricuspid Valve Disorders

- **Tricuspid Stenosis (TS)**: Rare, usually due to rheumatic fever or carcinoid syndrome.
  - Murmur: Diastolic rumble at the left lower sternal border.
  - Management: Valve replacement in severe cases.

- **Tricuspid Regurgitation (TR)**:
  - Commonly secondary to right ventricular dilation (functional TR).
  - Murmur: Holosystolic murmur best heard at the left lower sternal border, increases with

inspiration (Carvallo's sign).
- Management: Treat the underlying cause; surgery if severe.

Pearl:
- Severe functional TR often improves with correction of left-sided heart disease.

2. Pulmonary Valve Disorders
- **Pulmonary Stenosis (PS):**
    - Usually congenital.
    - Murmur: Harsh systolic ejection murmur at the left upper sternal border with ejection click.
    - Management: Balloon valvuloplasty for severe PS.
- **Pulmonary Regurgitation (PR):**
    - Secondary to pulmonary hypertension, endocarditis, or congenital heart disease repair.
    - Murmur: Early diastolic decrescendo murmur at the left upper sternal border.
    - Management: Rarely requires intervention unless symptomatic.

Pearl:
- PR is commonly asymptomatic and well-tolerated in most cases.

Surgical And Transcatheter Interventions

Surgical Interventions
- Indications depend on symptom severity, valve

anatomy, and impact on cardiac function.
- Valve repair is often preferred over replacement for mitral and tricuspid valves.

Transcatheter Interventions
- **TAVR**: Transformative for high-risk patients with severe AS.
- **MitraClip**: Minimally invasive option for severe symptomatic MR not amenable to surgery.
- **Percutaneous Balloon Valvuloplasty**: Preferred for MS and certain cases of PS.

Pearl:
- For patients with high surgical risk, transcatheter options have revolutionized the management of valvular heart disease, improving outcomes and reducing recovery times.

CHAPTER 5: ARRHYTHMIAS

Arrhythmias are a diverse group of conditions characterized by abnormal heart rhythms that can range from benign to life-threatening.

Supraventricular Tachycardia (Svt)

SVT encompasses a range of tachyarrhythmias originating above the ventricles, often causing palpitations and rapid heart rates.

Key Types:

1. **Atrioventricular Nodal Reentrant Tachycardia (AVNRT)**: Most common.
2. **Atrioventricular Reentrant Tachycardia (AVRT)**: Includes Wolff-Parkinson-White (WPW) syndrome.
3. **Atrial Tachycardia**: Rare, often associated with structural heart disease.

Management:

- **Acute:**
    - Vagal maneuvers (e.g., carotid sinus massage, Valsalva).
    - Adenosine for rapid termination in hemodynamically stable patients.
- **Chronic:**
    - Beta-blockers or calcium channel blockers for prevention.
    - Catheter ablation for recurrent or drug-

refractory SVT.

Pearl:
- Avoid AV nodal-blocking agents in WPW syndrome with pre-excited atrial fibrillation due to the risk of ventricular fibrillation.

Atrial Fibrillation (Af)

AF is the most common sustained arrhythmia, associated with increased risks of stroke, heart failure, and mortality.

Rate vs. Rhythm Control:
- **Rate Control:**
    - Preferred in most patients.
    - Agents: Beta-blockers, calcium channel blockers (e.g., diltiazem, verapamil), digoxin (in heart failure).
- **Rhythm Control:**
    - Consider in younger patients, those with persistent symptoms, or failed rate control.
    - Agents: Antiarrhythmics (e.g., amiodarone, flecainide), catheter ablation.

Anticoagulation Tips Based on CHA_2DS_2-VASc Score:
- **CHA_2DS_2-VASc:** Assesses stroke risk in nonvalvular AF.
    - **C:** Congestive heart failure (1).
    - **H:** Hypertension (1).
    - **A_2:** Age ≥75 years (2).
    - **D:** Diabetes mellitus (1).
    - **S_2:** Prior stroke/TIA/thromboembolism (2).
    - **V:** Vascular disease (1).
    - **A:** Age 65–74 years (1).
    - **Sc:** Sex category (female) (1).

- Anticoagulation recommendations:
    - Score ≥2 (men) or ≥3 (women): Oral anticoagulation.
    - Score 1 (men) or 2 (women): Consider anticoagulation based on risk-benefit.

Pearl:
- Direct oral anticoagulants (DOACs) are preferred over warfarin for most patients, barring contraindications such as valvular AF.

Ventricular Arrhythmias

1. Ventricular Tachycardia (VT):

Sustained VT is a rapid rhythm originating from the ventricles, often associated with structural heart disease.

- **Management**:
  - Acute: Amiodarone or lidocaine for stable VT; synchronized cardioversion for unstable VT.
  - Long-term: ICD placement; antiarrhythmic drugs for recurrent VT.

Pearl:
- Monomorphic VT suggests a scar-related reentry (e.g., post-MI), while polymorphic VT is often ischemia-related or due to electrolyte abnormalities.

2. Ventricular Fibrillation (VF):

VF is chaotic ventricular activity leading to cardiac arrest.

- **Management**:
  - Immediate defibrillation.
  - Address reversible causes (e.g., myocardial ischemia, electrolyte disturbances).

Pearl:
- Survivors of VF typically require ICD placement to prevent recurrence.

Bradyarrhythmias

1. Atrioventricular (AV) Blocks:

- **First-degree AV block**: Prolonged PR interval (>200 ms), generally benign.
- **Second-degree AV block**:
  - **Mobitz Type I (Wenckebach)**: Progressive PR prolongation with dropped beats; often asymptomatic.
  - **Mobitz Type II**: Sudden dropped beats without PR prolongation; higher risk of progression to complete heart block.
- **Third-degree (Complete) Heart Block**: No conduction between atria and ventricles, requiring immediate pacemaker placement.

Pearl:

- Mobitz Type II and third-degree blocks are indications for permanent pacemaker implantation.

2. Sinus Node Dysfunction:

- Includes sinus bradycardia, sinus arrest, and tachy-brady syndrome.
- **Management**:
  - Pacemaker implantation for symptomatic bradycardia or pause-related syncope.

Device Therapy

1. Pacemaker Indications:
- Symptomatic bradycardia.
- High-grade AV block (Mobitz Type II or complete heart block).
- Sinus node dysfunction with symptomatic pauses.

Pearl:
- Dual-chamber pacemakers mimic normal atrioventricular conduction and are preferred in most cases.

2. Implantable Cardioverter-Defibrillator (ICD) Indications:
- Primary prevention:
    - Ischemic cardiomyopathy with EF ≤35% and NYHA Class II/III despite GDMT.
    - Nonischemic cardiomyopathy with EF ≤35% after 3 months of optimized therapy.
- Secondary prevention:
    - Survivors of VT/VF without reversible causes.

3. Cardiac Resynchronization Therapy (CRT):
- Indicated for heart failure patients with EF ≤35%, LBBB with QRS ≥150 ms, and NYHA Class II–IV symptoms despite GDMT.

Pearl:
- CRT improves symptoms and reduces mortality in selected heart failure patients with electrical dyssynchrony.

CHAPTER 6: HYPERTENSION

Hypertension is a leading modifiable risk factor for cardiovascular disease and premature mortality.

Primary vs. Secondary Hypertension
Primary (Essential) Hypertension
- Accounts for **90–95%** of cases.
- Multifactorial etiology: genetics, lifestyle factors (e.g., obesity, high salt intake, physical inactivity), and age-related vascular changes.
- Typically asymptomatic and diagnosed during routine screening.

Pearls:
- Ensure accurate blood pressure (BP) measurement:
  - Patient seated and rested for 5 minutes.
  - Arm supported at heart level.
  - No caffeine, exercise, or smoking within 30 minutes of measurement.

Secondary Hypertension
- Occurs due to an underlying, often reversible condition.
- Accounts for **5–10%** of cases.

Common Causes:
1. **Renal**: Chronic kidney disease, renovascular hypertension.
2. **Endocrine**:
   - Primary hyperaldosteronism (Conn's

syndrome).
- Pheochromocytoma.
- Cushing's syndrome.
- Thyroid or parathyroid disorders.
3. **Cardiovascular**: Coarctation of the aorta.
4. **Drug-induced**: NSAIDs, corticosteroids, oral contraceptives.
5. **Obstructive Sleep Apnea (OSA)**.

Pearls:
- Suspect secondary hypertension if:
    - Onset is before 30 years or after 55 years.
    - BP is resistant to ≥3 antihypertensive agents.
    - Presence of target organ damage disproportionate to BP levels.

Management Guidelines And Resistant Hypertension

General Approach
- Lifestyle modifications:
    - Weight loss (goal BMI: 20–25 kg/m^2).
    - Low-sodium, high-potassium diet (e.g., DASH diet).
    - Regular physical activity.
    - Limiting alcohol intake.

Pharmacologic Therapy
- **First-line agents** (as per major guidelines like ACC/AHA, ESC/ESH):
    1. **ACE inhibitors (e.g., lisinopril)** or **ARBs (e.g., losartan)**: Preferred in diabetics and those with heart failure or chronic kidney disease.
    2. **Calcium channel blockers (e.g., amlodipine)**: Effective in the elderly and Black populations.
    3. **Thiazide diuretics (e.g., chlorthalidone)**: Effective for volume control.
- **Second-line agents**:
    - Beta-blockers (e.g., metoprolol) for those with specific indications (e.g., post-MI, heart failure).
    - Aldosterone antagonists (e.g., spironolactone) for resistant hypertension.

Resistant Hypertension
Defined as BP above target despite optimal doses of ≥**3 drugs** (including a diuretic).

Evaluation and Management:
- Rule out secondary causes.
- Ensure medication adherence and proper BP measurement.
- Add spironolactone or consider other agents like alpha-blockers (e.g., doxazosin).

Pearl:
- Always assess for "white coat hypertension" with home or ambulatory BP monitoring.

Hypertensive Emergencies

Hypertensive emergencies are characterized by severe BP elevation (≥180/120 mmHg) with evidence of acute target organ damage (e.g., encephalopathy, stroke, myocardial infarction, acute kidney injury).

Common Presentations:
1. **Hypertensive encephalopathy**: Headache, confusion, visual disturbances, seizures.
2. **Acute coronary syndrome**: Chest pain, ST changes.
3. **Acute heart failure**: Dyspnea, pulmonary edema.
4. **Aortic dissection**: Sudden tearing chest or back pain.
5. **Acute kidney injury**: Oliguria, elevated creatinine.

Management Tips:
- **Goal**: Reduce BP by no more than **25%** within the first hour to prevent ischemia.
    - Use **intravenous agents**:
        - **Nicardipine** or **clevidipine** for most cases.
        - **Nitroglycerin** for acute coronary syndromes or pulmonary edema.
        - **Esmolol** or **labetalol** for aortic

dissection.
- Monitor for signs of hypoperfusion or worsening organ function.

Hypertensive Urgencies:
- Severe BP elevation **without** acute organ damage.
- **Management**: Gradual BP reduction over 24–48 hours with oral agents (e.g., amlodipine, labetalol).

Pearls:
- Avoid overly rapid BP reduction to prevent ischemic complications (e.g., stroke, acute kidney injury).
- Always consider reversible triggers (e.g., medication nonadherence, pain, or substance use).

CHAPTER 7: CONGENITAL HEART DISEASES (ADULTS)

Congenital heart diseases (CHDs) are structural heart abnormalities that are present at birth. While many of these conditions are diagnosed in childhood, some patients may not experience symptoms until adulthood or may have symptoms that are mild and overlooked.

Atrial Septal Defect (Asd)

An **ASD** is a congenital hole in the wall (septum) that divides the left and right atria of the heart. It is one of the most common congenital heart defects, and its impact on adult patients often depends on the size of the defect and whether other cardiac abnormalities are present.

Types

1. **Ostium Secundum**: The most common type, located in the middle part of the septum.
2. **Ostium Primum**: Occurs lower in the septum and is often associated with other anomalies (e.g., cleft mitral valve).
3. **Sinus Venosus**: Involves the upper portion of the septum near the junction of the superior vena cava and right atrium.

Clinical Features

- Small to moderate ASDs may remain asymptomatic until later in life.
- Larger defects may cause **right-sided heart failure** symptoms, fatigue, and exercise intolerance due to increased right atrial and ventricular volume overload.

- **Paradoxical embolism**: A risk for stroke, where blood clots from the venous circulation pass into the arterial circulation through the ASD.

Diagnosis
- **Echocardiography**: The gold standard for diagnosis, including transesophageal echocardiography (TEE) for better visualization of the defect.
- **Bubble study**: Used to assess for a shunt between the atria.
- **Cardiac MRI**: Can provide a detailed assessment in complex cases.

Management Pearls
- **Closure indications**:
  - Symptomatic patients.
  - Evidence of right heart enlargement.
  - Presence of paradoxical embolism.
- **Device closure**: Percutaneous closure with an occluder device is increasingly common, offering a less invasive alternative to surgery.
- **Surgical closure**: Recommended for large defects or when percutaneous closure is not feasible.

Ventricular Septal Defect (Vsd)

A **VSD** *is a congenital opening in the interventricular septum, the wall that separates the left and right ventricles. It is the most common congenital heart defect diagnosed in childhood.*

Types
1. **Perimembranous**: The most common type, located near the aortic valve.
2. **Muscular**: Located in the lower part of the septum, often multiple and may close spontaneously in

childhood.
3. **Inlet**: Located near the tricuspid and mitral valves.
4. **Outlet**: Near the pulmonary valve, less common.

Clinical Features

- **Small to moderate VSDs** may be asymptomatic, but larger defects lead to **left-to-right shunting** and right-sided heart failure.
- **Symptoms** in adults include dyspnea, fatigue, and exercise intolerance due to increased pulmonary blood flow and eventual pulmonary hypertension.
- **Harsh holosystolic murmur** is commonly heard at the left lower sternal border.

Diagnosis

- **Echocardiography**: The primary diagnostic tool, with Doppler flow studies to assess the degree of shunting and potential complications like pulmonary hypertension.
- **Cardiac MRI or CT**: In complex cases, these can provide detailed anatomic information.

Management Pearls

- **Small defects**: May not require intervention and can be followed with regular monitoring.
- **Moderate to large VSDs**: Surgical or device closure may be necessary, especially if there is evidence of pulmonary hypertension or significant left-to-right shunting.
- **Pulmonary hypertension**: If present, the defect may require closure sooner to prevent progression to Eisenmenger syndrome.

Tetralogy Of Fallot (Tof)

Tetralogy of Fallot (TOF) is one of the most common congenital cyanotic heart diseases.

It consists of a combination of four cardiac anomalies:
1. **Ventricular septal defect (VSD)**.
2. **Pulmonary stenosis**: Narrowing of the pulmonary outflow tract.
3. **Right ventricular hypertrophy (RVH)**: Thickening of the right ventricle due to the increased workload.
4. **Overriding aorta**: The aorta is displaced over the VSD, receiving blood from both ventricles.

Clinical Features
- **Cyanosis**: Due to right-to-left shunting through the VSD and underdevelopment of the pulmonary circulation.
- **"Tet spells"**: Episodes of deep cyanosis, often triggered by crying or exertion, leading to hypoxemia and requiring squatting in children to increase systemic vascular resistance.
- **Heart murmur**: Typically a systolic ejection murmur due to the pulmonary stenosis.

Diagnosis
- **Echocardiography**: Essential for evaluating the anatomy of the defects.
- **Chest X-ray**: Shows the characteristic "boot-shaped" heart due to right ventricular hypertrophy.
- **Cardiac MRI or CT**: Can be used for complex cases or pre-surgical planning.

Management Pearls

- **Surgical repair**: Involves closure of the VSD and relief of the right ventricular outflow tract obstruction, typically performed in infancy or early childhood.
- **Long-term follow-up**: Many adults with TOF will require follow-up for complications such as **pulmonary regurgitation** or **arrhythmias**, and some may need **pulmonary valve replacement** later in life.
- **Endocarditis prophylaxis**: Should be considered for patients with a history of uncorrected TOF or residual defects.

Eisenmenger Syndrome

*Eisenmenger syndrome is a condition in which a congenital **left-to-right shunt** (e.g., from ASD or VSD) causes long-standing pulmonary overload, leading to **pulmonary hypertension**. Over time, the pulmonary vascular resistance increases, and the shunt becomes **right-to-left**, causing **cyanosis** and complications of **hypoxemia**.*

Pathophysiology
- The initial left-to-right shunt results in increased pulmonary blood flow, leading to endothelial injury and remodeling of the pulmonary vasculature.
- Over time, the elevated pulmonary pressure results in a reversal of the shunt, and **cyanotic heart disease** develops, marked by **hypoxemia** and **polycythemia**.

Clinical Features
- **Cyanosis**: A hallmark sign due to right-to-left shunting.
- **Clubbing**: Common in adults with Eisenmenger syndrome due to chronic hypoxia.
- **Polycythemia**: Secondary to chronic hypoxemia, leading to an increased risk of thromboembolic events.
- **Shortness of breath**, **fatigue**, and **syncope**.

Diagnosis
- **Echocardiography**: To assess the shunt and pulmonary pressures.
- **Right heart catheterization**: The gold standard for diagnosing pulmonary hypertension and assessing the direction of shunting.

Management Pearls

- **No surgical closure**: In Eisenmenger syndrome, closing the shunt is not recommended due to the risk of precipitating right heart failure.
- **Pulmonary vasodilators**: Medications like **prostacyclin analogs** or **endothelin receptor antagonists** may be considered to manage pulmonary hypertension.
- **Oxygen therapy**: Long-term oxygen may be needed to alleviate hypoxemia.
- **Avoid high-altitude environments**: To reduce the risk of severe hypoxemia.
- **Thromboprophylaxis**: Due to the increased risk of thromboembolism from polycythemia.

CHAPTER 8: CARDIOMYOPATHIES

Cardiomyopathies are a group of diseases that affect the heart muscle, leading to structural and functional abnormalities.

They can result in heart failure, arrhythmias, and sudden cardiac death. Understanding the different types of cardiomyopathies— **dilated**, **hypertrophic**, **restrictive**, *and* **arrhythmogenic**—*is essential for effective management and risk stratification.*

Additionally, genetic testing and family screening are important tools in diagnosing and managing these conditions, particularly since many cardiomyopathies are inherited.

Dilated Cardiomyopathy (Dcm)

Dilated cardiomyopathy (DCM) *is characterized by* **ventricular dilation** *and impaired contraction of the heart muscle.*

The heart becomes enlarged, and its ability to pump blood efficiently is reduced, often leading to **heart failure** *with* **reduced ejection fraction (HFrEF)**.

Etiology

- **Idiopathic**: In many cases, the exact cause is unknown.
- **Genetic**: Mutations in genes encoding for sarcomere proteins or structural components of the heart muscle are common.
- **Infectious**: Viral myocarditis, particularly from **Coxsackievirus B**, can lead to DCM.

- **Toxic**: Alcohol, cocaine, or chemotherapy drugs (e.g., **doxorubicin**) can cause DCM.
- **Metabolic**: Conditions like **hypothyroidism**, **diabetes**, and **iron overload** (hemochromatosis) are potential causes.
- **Pregnancy**: **Peripartum cardiomyopathy** occurs in the late stages of pregnancy or within months after childbirth.

Clinical Features
- Symptoms of heart failure, including **dyspnea**, **fatigue**, **edema**, and **orthopnea**.
- **Systolic murmur**: Due to mitral regurgitation from left ventricular dilation.
- **Arrhythmias**: Risk of **atrial fibrillation** and **ventricular arrhythmias**.
- **Sudden cardiac death (SCD)**: A major concern, especially in younger individuals with genetic forms of DCM.

Diagnosis
- **Echocardiography**: Reveals **ventricular dilation**, **decreased ejection fraction**, and mitral regurgitation.
- **Cardiac MRI**: Provides detailed assessment of myocardial fibrosis and infarction.
- **Endomyocardial biopsy**: May be needed in suspected cases of myocarditis or infiltrative diseases.

Management Pearls
- **Heart failure management**: ACE inhibitors, **beta-blockers**, **diuretics**, and **aldosterone antagonists**.
- **Anticoagulation**: In the presence of atrial fibrillation

or large thrombus formation in the left ventricle.
- **Device therapy**: **Implantable cardioverter-defibrillators (ICD)** for primary prevention of sudden cardiac death, **cardiac resynchronization therapy (CRT)** in patients with heart failure and conduction delay.
- **Heart transplantation**: Considered in advanced cases of heart failure unresponsive to medical therapy.

Hypertrophic Cardiomyopathy (Hcm)

*Hypertrophic cardiomyopathy (HCM) is a condition where the heart muscle becomes **thickened**, most often affecting the **left ventricle**.*

The thickening can obstruct the outflow of blood and impair the heart's ability to pump effectively. It is one of the most common causes of sudden cardiac death in young athletes.

Etiology

- **Genetic**: HCM is primarily caused by mutations in **sarcomeric proteins** (e.g., **MYH7**, **MYBPC3**), following an **autosomal dominant inheritance pattern**.
- **Idiopathic**: In many cases, the cause is unknown, though genetic testing can often identify underlying mutations.

Clinical Features

- **Chest pain**, **dyspnea**, and **syncope** are common due to impaired ventricular filling, left ventricular outflow tract obstruction, and arrhythmias.
- **Systolic murmur**: Increased intensity with **valsalva maneuver** (due to outflow tract obstruction).
- **Palpitations**: Due to arrhythmias, including **atrial fibrillation** and **ventricular arrhythmias**.
- **Sudden cardiac death (SCD)**: Often occurs during exertion due to **ventricular arrhythmias**.

Diagnosis

- **Echocardiography**: Identifies asymmetric septal hypertrophy and outflow tract obstruction.
- **Cardiac MRI**: Can provide a more precise assessment of

the hypertrophy and any scarring.
- **Electrocardiogram (ECG)**: May show **left ventricular hypertrophy** (LVH), **atrial fibrillation**, or **Q waves**.

Management Pearls

- **Beta-blockers**: First-line therapy for symptom control, particularly for exercise intolerance and chest pain.
- **Calcium channel blockers**: Used in cases where beta-blockers are not effective.
- **Disopyramide**: For patients with significant symptoms related to obstruction.
- **Surgical intervention**: **Septal myectomy** (surgical reduction of hypertrophic septum) may be required in cases of significant outflow tract obstruction.
- **Alcohol septal ablation**: A less invasive alternative to myectomy.
- **ICD implantation**: For patients at high risk of sudden cardiac death, particularly those with a family history of SCD.

Restrictive Cardiomyopathy (Rcm)

*Restrictive cardiomyopathy (RCM) is characterized by **diastolic dysfunction** with preserved systolic function.*
The heart muscle becomes stiff and less able to expand during diastole, leading to impaired filling of the ventricles.

Etiology

- **Idiopathic**: The most common form in developed countries.
- **Infiltrative diseases**: Conditions such as **amyloidosis**, **sarcoidosis**, and **hemochromatosis** can lead to

restrictive cardiomyopathy.
- **Fibrotic diseases**: Conditions like **radiation therapy** or **endomyocardial fibrosis**.

Clinical Features

- **Heart failure** symptoms, particularly **right-sided heart failure** (e.g., **edema, ascites, jugular venous distension**).
- **Diastolic murmur**: Due to impaired ventricular filling.
- **Fatigue, exercise intolerance**, and **syncope** are common.

Diagnosis

- **Echocardiography**: Shows **normal systolic function, bi-atrial enlargement**, and **diastolic dysfunction**.
- **Cardiac MRI**: Can help assess the extent of fibrosis or infiltration.
- **Endomyocardial biopsy**: Useful in diagnosing amyloidosis and other infiltrative diseases.

Management Pearls

- **Heart failure management**: Standard heart failure therapies such as **ACE inhibitors, diuretics**, and **beta-blockers**.
- **Infiltrative disease treatment**: For example, **chelation therapy** for hemochromatosis or **chemotherapy** for amyloidosis.
- **Heart transplantation**: May be the ultimate treatment for advanced restrictive cardiomyopathy, especially in cases of severe heart failure.

Arrhythmogenic Right Ventricular Cardiomyopathy (Arvc)

*Arrhythmogenic right ventricular cardiomyopathy (ARVC) is a rare genetic condition characterized by the replacement of **right ventricular myocardium** with **fibrofatty tissue**, leading to **right ventricular dysfunction** and arrhythmias.*

Etiology

- **Genetic**: Caused by mutations in desmosomal proteins (e.g., **PKP2, DSP, DSG2**).
- **Inheritance**: Autosomal dominant.

Clinical Features

- **Arrhythmias**: Particularly **ventricular tachycardia** (VT), originating from the right ventricle. Syncope or sudden cardiac death may occur.
- **Right heart failure** symptoms such as **edema** and **ascites**.
- **Palpitations** due to arrhythmias.

Diagnosis

- **Electrocardiogram (ECG)**: Shows **inverted T waves** and **epsilon waves** (late potentials) in the right precordial leads.
- **Echocardiography**: Right ventricular dilation and dysfunction.
- **Cardiac MRI**: Can assess the extent of **fibrofatty replacement** of the right ventricle.

Management Pearls

- **ICD implantation**: Essential for prevention of sudden cardiac death.
- **Antiarrhythmic therapy**: Beta-blockers and **sodium channel blockers** may be used for arrhythmia control.
- **Heart transplantation**: Considered in advanced cases with severe right heart failure.

Genetic Testing And Family Screening

*Many cardiomyopathies have a **genetic basis**, making genetic testing and family screening essential for diagnosis, management, and risk stratification.*

Genetic Testing

- **Indications**:
    - Patients with early-onset cardiomyopathy.
    - Family history of sudden cardiac death or cardiomyopathy.
    - Diagnosis of a suspected inherited cardiomyopathy.
- **Targeted testing**: Genetic testing can identify mutations in genes encoding sarcomeric proteins or desmosomal components. This can help confirm the diagnosis and guide management decisions, particularly for patients with **HCM** or **DCM**.
- **Clinical utility**: Genetic testing can also provide information on prognosis and the likelihood of disease progression.

Family Screening

- **First-degree relatives** of affected individuals should undergo screening to identify those at risk,

particularly in inherited forms of cardiomyopathy.
- Screening typically includes **ECG**, **echocardiography**, and possibly **genetic testing** to detect early signs of the condition.
- Early detection allows for **preventive interventions**, such as **ICD placement** or lifestyle modifications to reduce the risk of sudden cardiac death.

Pearls for Genetic Counseling
- **Autosomal dominant inheritance** means that each child of an affected individual has a 50% chance of inheriting the disease.
- **Prenatal testing** may be available for families with known genetic mutations.
- Genetic counseling is essential for patients and families to understand the implications of testing and family screening.

CHAPTER 9: INFECTIVE ENDOCARDITIS AND RHEUMATIC HEART DISEASE

Infective endocarditis (IE) and rheumatic heart disease (RHD) are two important cardiac conditions that have distinct causes but share similar complications, including valve damage and systemic embolism.

Both conditions require timely diagnosis and appropriate management to prevent severe outcomes, such as heart failure, stroke, or death.

Infective Endocarditis (Ie)

Infective endocarditis is an infection of the endocardium, typically involving the heart valves.

It can occur when bacteria or fungi enter the bloodstream and attach to damaged or prosthetic heart valves.

*The infection leads to the formation of **vegetations**—masses of platelets, fibrin, microorganisms, and inflammatory cells—on the heart valves.*

Duke's Criteria for Diagnosis of Infective Endocarditis

The diagnosis of infective endocarditis is made using the **Duke Criteria**, which are divided into **major** and **minor** criteria.

The diagnosis is confirmed when there are either:

- **Two major criteria**, or
- **One major criterion and three minor criteria**, or
- **Five minor criteria**.

Major Criteria

1. **Positive blood cultures**: Blood cultures drawn from at least three separate sites showing growth of microorganisms typically associated with endocarditis, such as **Staphylococcus aureus**, **Streptococcus viridans**, or **Enterococcus**.
    - **Persistent bacteremia**: Blood cultures positive for the same organism on two separate occasions, or persistent bacteremia despite appropriate antimicrobial therapy.
2. **Evidence of endocardial involvement**: This includes findings such as:
    - **Echocardiographic evidence** of a vegetation, abscess, or prosthetic valve dysfunction.
    - New valvular regurgitation (e.g., **mitral** or **aortic regurgitation**).

Minor Criteria

1. **Predisposing heart conditions or intravenous drug use**.
2. **Fever**: A temperature greater than 38°C (100.4°F).
3. **Vascular phenomena**: Including **embolism, Janeway lesions, roth spots**, or **splinter hemorrhages**.
4. **Immunologic phenomena**: Such as **Osler's nodes, glomerulonephritis**, or **positive rheumatoid factor**.
5. **Microbiological evidence**: Positive blood cultures that do not meet the major criteria (e.g., single positive

blood culture for a microorganism that is less likely to cause endocarditis).

Clinical Features of Infective Endocarditis

- **Fever**: Often the most prominent symptom, though it may be absent in older adults or those with prosthetic valves.
- **Heart murmurs**: New or worsening murmurs, particularly regurgitant murmurs.
- **Embolic phenomena: Stroke, splenic infarction**, or **renal infarction** can occur due to embolization of vegetations.
- **Signs of heart failure**: Due to valvular dysfunction or septic embolism.
- **Petechiae**: Small purple spots on the skin, mucous membranes, or conjunctiva.
- **Splinter hemorrhages**: Small, linear blood clots under the nails.

Management of Infective Endocarditis

- **Antibiotics**: Empiric antibiotic therapy is started immediately after blood cultures are drawn, typically with **ceftriaxone**, **vancomycin**, or **daptomycin**, depending on local resistance patterns. The antibiotic regimen is then adjusted based on culture results.
- **Duration**: Antibiotic therapy usually lasts for **4-6 weeks**, depending on the severity and pathogen.
- **Surgical treatment**: Surgical intervention is indicated for:
  - **Severe valve dysfunction** causing heart failure.
  - **Uncontrolled infection** despite antibiotics.

- **Large vegetations** at risk for embolism.
- **Prosthetic valve endocarditis**.

Antibiotic Prophylaxis for Endocarditis

Certain patients are at increased risk for infective endocarditis, particularly those with prosthetic heart valves, previous history of infective endocarditis, or specific congenital heart conditions. ***Antibiotic prophylaxis*** *is recommended in these high-risk patients before certain procedures, such as dental procedures or surgeries, that may introduce bacteria into the bloodstream.*

Indications For Prophylaxis

- **Prosthetic heart valves** or **prosthetic material** used in heart valve repair.
- **History of infective endocarditis**.
- **Congenital heart disease**:
  - **Unrepaired cyanotic congenital heart disease**.
  - **Completely repaired congenital heart defect** with prosthetic material or device for the first six months post-repair.
  - **Cardiac transplant recipients** who develop valvulopathy.
- **Dental procedures**: Especially those involving **manipulation of the gums** or **root canal therapy**.

Regimen: Typically, **amoxicillin** (or **clindamycin** for penicillin-allergic patients) is given 30-60 minutes before the procedure.

Rheumatic Heart Disease (Rhd)

*Rheumatic heart disease is a complication of **rheumatic fever**, a condition that arises after an **acute group A streptococcal throat infection**.*

*The immune response to the infection leads to inflammation in various tissues, including the heart, joints, and skin. When the inflammation affects the heart, it can lead to **valvular damage**, particularly the **mitral valve**.*

Pathophysiology of Rheumatic Heart Disease

- **Acute phase**: The immune system mistakenly targets the body's own tissues, leading to **mitral valve regurgitation** (the most common valvular involvement), and potentially **aortic valve involvement**.
- **Chronic phase**: Repeated episodes of rheumatic fever result in **scarring** and **thickening** of the heart valves, leading to **mitral stenosis**, **mitral regurgitation**, or **aortic stenosis**.

Clinical Features

- **Carditis**: Inflammation of the heart, which may present with **murmurs** (mitral or aortic valve involvement).
- **Arthritis**: Migratory polyarthritis is one of the hallmark features of acute rheumatic fever.
- **Erythema marginatum**: A characteristic rash with raised red edges and a pale center.
- **Sydenham chorea**: A neurologic manifestation involving involuntary movements.

Diagnosis

- **Jones Criteria**: The diagnosis of rheumatic fever requires the presence of **two major criteria** or **one major and two minor criteria**, in addition to evidence of a recent streptococcal infection (e.g., positive throat culture or **antistreptolysin O (ASO)** titer).
    - **Major criteria**: Includes **carditis, arthritis, chorea, erythema marginatum**, and **subcutaneous nodules**.
    - **Minor criteria**: Includes **fever, arthralgia**, and **elevated acute-phase reactants** (e.g., ESR, CRP).

Management of Rheumatic Heart Disease

- **Antibiotics**: Penicillin is given to eliminate any remaining streptococcal infection and to prevent recurrence of rheumatic fever.
- **Anti-inflammatory treatment**: **Aspirin** or **corticosteroids** can help manage inflammation, particularly for arthritis and carditis.
- **Valve repair or replacement**: In cases of severe valvular damage (e.g., **mitral stenosis** or **mitral regurgitation**), surgery may be required.
- **Secondary prevention**: Long-term prophylaxis with **penicillin** or **azithromycin** to prevent recurrent streptococcal infections and further valve damage.

Complications And Surgical Indications For Infective Endocarditis And Rheumatic Heart Disease

Both infective endocarditis and rheumatic heart disease can lead to serious complications, including **heart failure, embolic events**, and **valvular deformities**.

Complications Of Infective Endocarditis

- **Heart failure**: Due to valve dysfunction or severe infection.
- **Embolic events**: Stroke, renal infarction, and splenic infarction due to the embolization of vegetations.
- **Abscess formation**: Can develop within the heart or other organs.
- **Persistent bacteremia**: Leading to septic shock and multi-organ failure.

Surgical Indications In Endocarditis

- **Severe valve dysfunction**: Leading to heart failure that is refractory to medical therapy.
- **Prosthetic valve endocarditis**: Particularly if complicated by abscess formation or persistent infection despite antibiotic therapy.
- **Large vegetations**: With a high risk of embolism.
- **Uncontrolled infection**: If the infection cannot be eradicated with antibiotics alone.

Complications of Rheumatic Heart Disease

- **Heart failure**: Due to mitral or aortic valve disease.
- **Arrhythmias**: **Atrial fibrillation** is common in patients with long-standing mitral stenosis.
- **Systemic embolism**: From thrombus formation in the left atrium (particularly in mitral stenosis).

Surgical Indications in Rheumatic Heart Disease

- **Severe valvular stenosis** or regurgitation: Requiring valve repair or replacement, typically with **mechanical**

or **bioprosthetic** valves.
- **Mitral valve replacement**: Indicated in patients with severe mitral stenosis or regurgitation who are symptomatic or have heart failure.

CHAPTER 11: CARDIAC IMAGING AND DIAGNOSTICS

Cardiac imaging and diagnostic tests are critical tools in the evaluation and management of patients with suspected or known cardiovascular conditions.

Understanding the indications, techniques, and interpretation of these tests is essential for making accurate diagnoses and guiding appropriate management.

Ecg: Quick Pearls For Common Findings

The electrocardiogram (ECG) is one of the most frequently used tools in cardiology for diagnosing arrhythmias, ischemia, and other cardiac abnormalities. Understanding key findings on the ECG can significantly impact clinical decision-making.

- **ST-Elevation Myocardial Infarction (STEMI):**
    - **Pearl**: Look for new, prominent **ST-segment elevation** (greater than 1 mm in two contiguous leads) in the **precordial** and **limb leads**, which strongly suggests acute transmural ischemia.
    - **Action**: Immediate **reperfusion therapy** (PCI or fibrinolysis) should be considered based on time of presentation.
- **Atrial Fibrillation (AF):**
    - **Pearl**: The absence of distinct **P waves** with an irregularly irregular rhythm suggests atrial fibrillation.
    - **Action**: Rate control (e.g., **beta-blockers**

or **calcium channel blockers**) and anticoagulation based on the **CHA2DS2-VASc score** are essential in management.

- **Bradyarrhythmias (e.g., Sinus Bradycardia and AV Block):**
  - **Pearl:** Look for a **long PR interval** (>300 ms) indicating **first-degree AV block** or a **second-degree block** with dropped beats (Mobitz Type I or II).
  - **Action:** Depending on symptoms, pacemaker placement may be necessary for patients with symptomatic bradyarrhythmias.
- **T-wave Inversion:**
  - **Pearl: T-wave inversion** in the lateral leads (I, aVL, V5, and V6) could suggest ischemia, especially in the setting of chest pain.
  - **Action:** Consider **cardiac biomarkers** and **coronary angiography** if ischemia is suspected.
- **Ventricular Tachycardia (VT):**
  - **Pearl:** A **wide QRS complex** with a **monomorphic** pattern is highly suggestive of VT, particularly if associated with hemodynamic instability.
  - **Action:** Immediate **electrical cardioversion** is required if the patient is unstable. If stable, **antiarrhythmic drugs** (e.g., **amiodarone**) may be used.

Echocardiography: Key Indications And Interpretation Tips

Echocardiography is a non-invasive imaging technique that provides real-time visualization of cardiac structures and function. It is crucial for evaluating heart chambers, valves, and ventricular function.

- **Indications**:
    - **Chest Pain**: For suspected ischemic heart disease, **stress echocardiography** can help assess wall motion abnormalities during exercise or pharmacologic stress.
    - **Heart Failure: Echocardiography** is essential for differentiating between **HFrEF** (Heart Failure with reduced ejection fraction) and **HFpEF** (Heart Failure with preserved ejection fraction).
    - **Valvular Heart Disease**: A comprehensive **transthoracic echocardiogram (TTE)** can assess valve structure, function, and the presence of stenosis or regurgitation.
    - **Endocarditis**: **Transesophageal echocardiography (TEE)** is highly sensitive for detecting **vegetations** in infective endocarditis, especially in prosthetic valves or difficult-to-visualize areas.
- **Interpretation Pearls**:
    - **Left Ventricular Ejection Fraction (LVEF)**: Measures the percentage of blood pumped out of the left ventricle with each heartbeat. An LVEF less than 40% suggests significant systolic dysfunction.
    - **Mitral Regurgitation (MR)**: Look for a **holosystolic murmur** and **jet** on Doppler imaging to assess severity. Severe MR may require surgical intervention.
    - **Aortic Stenosis (AS)**: Measure the **aortic valve area** and assess the **velocity** of the jet across the valve. A valve area less than 1 cm^2

usually warrants consideration for surgery.
- **Pericardial Effusion**: Evaluate the size of the effusion and the presence of **diastolic collapse** of the right atrium and ventricle, which may indicate **cardiac tamponade**.

Cardiac Mri And Ct: When To Order

*Both **Cardiac MRI (CMR)** and **Cardiac CT (CCT)** provide detailed imaging for specific indications, particularly when echocardiography cannot provide sufficient information.*

- **Cardiac MRI**:
  - **Indications**:
    - **Myocardial Scar Assessment**: CMR is ideal for assessing **fibrosis** or **scarring** post-myocardial infarction.
    - **Cardiomyopathies**: CMR can assess **wall motion abnormalities**, **ventricular dilation**, and **fibrosis** in **dilated cardiomyopathy** or **hypertrophic cardiomyopathy**.
    - **Pericardial Disease**: CMR is the gold standard for evaluating **pericardial thickness** and **constrictive pericarditis**.
  - **Pearl: Late gadolinium enhancement** on CMR is highly sensitive for detecting areas of myocardial infarction and scar tissue.
- **Cardiac CT**:
  - **Indications**:
    - **Coronary Artery Disease (CAD)**: Cardiac CT angiography (CTA) is useful in the evaluation of coronary

artery anatomy, particularly for non-invasive coronary artery assessment.
- **Aortic Pathologies**: CCT is the gold standard for evaluating aortic dissections, aneurysms, and congenital aortic anomalies.
- **Valve Assessment**: CCT can provide detailed imaging for **aortic valve** pathology or **mitral valve** calcification, which can affect surgical planning.

◦ **Pearl**: **Coronary CTA** should be used in low- to intermediate-risk patients with chest pain to avoid invasive angiography.

CHAPTER 12: PREVENTIVE CARDIOLOGY

Preventive cardiology focuses on reducing the risk of cardiovascular diseases (CVD) before they occur.

The goal is to prevent heart attacks, strokes, and other cardiovascular events through early identification of risk factors, aggressive management of modifiable risk factors, and lifestyle interventions.

Lipid Management: Statins, Pcsk9 Inhibitors, And Beyond

The management of cholesterol levels plays a crucial role in the prevention of atherosclerotic cardiovascular disease (ASCVD), which includes coronary artery disease, stroke, and peripheral artery disease.

Here are key interventions for lipid management:

- **Statins**:
    - **Pearl**: Statins are the first-line therapy for managing **low-density lipoprotein cholesterol (LDL-C)** and reducing cardiovascular risk. They reduce LDL-C by blocking the enzyme **HMG-CoA reductase**, which is involved in cholesterol synthesis.
    - **High-Intensity Statins**: For patients at high risk of cardiovascular events (e.g., those with a history of heart attack or stroke), high-intensity statins (e.g., **atorvastatin 40–80 mg** or **rosuvastatin 20–40 mg**) should be used to

- lower LDL-C by 50% or more.
  - **Moderate-Intensity Statins**: For those with lower risk, moderate-intensity statins (e.g., **simvastatin 20–40 mg**) are often sufficient.
- **PCSK9 Inhibitors**:
  - **Pearl**: **PCSK9 inhibitors** (e.g., **alirocumab, evolocumab**) are monoclonal antibodies that increase the liver's ability to clear LDL-C from the blood by inhibiting the **PCSK9 enzyme**, which normally reduces LDL receptors on liver cells.
  - **Indications**: PCSK9 inhibitors are used in patients with **familial hypercholesterolemia**, those with high **cardiovascular risk** who do not achieve adequate LDL-C reduction with statins alone, or those who are statin-intolerant.
  - **Benefits**: These agents can lower LDL-C by up to 60%, significantly reducing the risk of heart attack, stroke, and death from cardiovascular causes.
- **Ezetimibe**:
  - **Pearl**: **Ezetimibe** is a cholesterol absorption inhibitor that reduces cholesterol absorption in the small intestine. It is typically used in combination with statins for further LDL-C lowering, especially in patients who do not reach their LDL-C targets with statins alone.
  - **Indications**: It may be added when patients are at high risk or those who do not achieve adequate LDL-C reductions with statin monotherapy.
- **Bempedoic Acid**:

- **Pearl**: Bempedoic acid is an alternative option for lowering LDL-C, working by inhibiting ATP citrate lyase (ACL), an enzyme involved in cholesterol production. It is typically used when statins and other agents are not sufficient or well-tolerated.
- **Indications**: It can be used in combination with statins or as an alternative in statin-intolerant patients.

Lifestyle Interventions: Diet, Exercise, And Smoking Cessation

While pharmacologic interventions are crucial in reducing cardiovascular risk, lifestyle modifications are the cornerstone of preventive cardiology.

Patients should be encouraged to adopt healthy behaviors to improve heart health.

- **Diet**:
  - **Pearl**: A heart-healthy diet rich in fruits, vegetables, whole grains, lean proteins, and healthy fats (e.g., from **olive oil** and **avocados**) can help reduce LDL-C levels, lower blood pressure, and reduce overall cardiovascular risk.
  - **Key Dietary Components**:
    - **Reduce saturated fats** found in red meat, butter, and full-fat dairy products.
    - **Increase fiber** by consuming more **fruits, vegetables, legumes**, and **whole grains**.

- **Increase omega-3 fatty acids** from sources like **fatty fish**, flaxseeds, and walnuts, which can help reduce triglycerides and inflammation.
- Limit **sodium intake** to less than 2,300 mg per day, or ideally 1,500 mg per day, to help lower blood pressure.

- **Exercise**:
  - **Pearl**: Regular physical activity, particularly **aerobic exercise**, is highly beneficial in reducing cardiovascular risk. It improves lipid profiles, lowers blood pressure, enhances endothelial function, and helps maintain a healthy weight.
  - **Recommendations**:
    - Adults should aim for at least **150 minutes** of moderate-intensity exercise (e.g., brisk walking, cycling) or **75 minutes** of vigorous-intensity exercise (e.g., running, swimming) per week.
    - Additionally, include **muscle-strengthening activities** at least twice a week.
    - **High-Intensity Interval Training (HIIT)** has also been shown to be effective in improving cardiovascular health in shorter durations.

- **Smoking Cessation**:
  - **Pearl**: Smoking is one of the most significant modifiable risk factors for CVD, contributing to the development of **atherosclerosis**, **endothelial dysfunction**, and **increased clotting risk**.

- **Intervention**: Smoking cessation should be strongly encouraged in all patients, with pharmacologic assistance (e.g., **nicotine replacement therapy**, **varenicline**, **bupropion**) offered to help patients quit.
- **Benefit**: Quitting smoking significantly reduces the risk of heart disease, with the risk approaching that of non-smokers within 1–2 years.

Screening In High-Risk Populations

Early detection of cardiovascular risk factors is key to preventing heart disease.

Screening should be tailored to individual risk profiles, with specific emphasis on high-risk populations.

- **Hypertension Screening**:
    - **Pearl**: Blood pressure should be measured at least once every two years in adults, with annual screenings in those at higher risk (e.g., overweight, family history of hypertension, or diabetes).
    - **Management**: Initiate lifestyle changes first, with pharmacologic treatment (e.g., **ACE inhibitors, diuretics, beta-blockers**) for those with stage 1 or higher hypertension.
- **Lipid Screening**:
    - **Pearl**: **Lipid panels** should be checked every 4–6 years starting at age 20 for all adults, and more frequently in high-risk patients (e.g., those with diabetes, a family history of early heart disease, or existing heart disease).
    - **High-Risk Populations**: Focus on early screening in **individuals with familial hypercholesterolemia, those with diabetes**, and **those with a family history** of early heart disease.
- **Diabetes Screening**:
    - **Pearl**: **Diabetes** is a significant risk factor for cardiovascular disease. Screen for type 2 diabetes with a fasting plasma glucose or hemoglobin A1c measurement in individuals

with risk factors (e.g., obesity, family history).
- **Management**: Good glucose control, achieved through diet, exercise, and medications (e.g., **metformin, GLP-1 receptor agonists**), is essential for reducing cardiovascular risk in diabetic patients.

- **Coronary Artery Calcium (CAC) Scoring**:
    - **Pearl**: **CAC scoring** is a non-invasive imaging technique that helps assess the risk of coronary artery disease (CAD), particularly in patients with intermediate risk. Higher CAC scores correlate with a higher risk of future cardiovascular events.
    - **Indications**: Consider in patients with a 10-year ASCVD risk between 5% and 20% who are uncertain about starting statins.

CHAPTER 13: CARDIOLOGY EMERGENCIES

Cardiology emergencies are critical situations that require prompt identification and management to prevent significant morbidity and mortality.

Acute Heart Failure And Cardiogenic Shock

Acute heart failure and cardiogenic shock are life-threatening conditions often precipitated by acute myocardial infarction (MI), severe arrhythmias, or chronic heart failure exacerbations.

- **Acute Heart Failure (AHF):**
    - **Pearl**: Rapid identification of **left ventricular dysfunction** (through clinical assessment and echocardiography) is essential. Common signs include **dyspnea**, **orthopnea**, and **pulmonary edema**.
    - **Management**: Initiate **oxygen therapy** and **diuretics** (e.g., **furosemide**) to reduce fluid overload. In some cases, **vasodilators** like **nitroglycerin** may be used to reduce preload and afterload. Consider **inotropes** like **dobutamine** if there is persistent low cardiac output despite fluid resuscitation.
- **Cardiogenic Shock**:
    - **Pearl**: The hallmark of cardiogenic shock is **hypotension** and **end-organ hypoperfusion** despite adequate intravascular volume. Most

commonly, it follows **acute MI** or severe left ventricular dysfunction.

- **Management**: **Inotropic support** (e.g., **dopamine**, **dobutamine**) and **mechanical circulatory support** (e.g., **intra-aortic balloon pump (IABP)** or **extracorporeal membrane oxygenation (ECMO)**) may be required for refractory shock. Prompt **reperfusion therapy** (e.g., **PCI** or **fibrinolysis**) is crucial in STEMI-related cardiogenic shock.

Acute Coronary Syndromes: Door-To-Balloon Tips

Timely reperfusion in acute coronary syndromes (ACS) is critical for minimizing myocardial damage and improving patient outcomes. The "door-to-balloon" time is a key performance metric in the management of STEMI.

- **Door-to-Balloon Time**:
    - **Pearl**: Aim for a door-to-balloon time of **<90 minutes** for STEMI patients requiring primary PCI.
    - **Action**: **Pre-hospital triage** and **early activation of the catheterization lab** can significantly reduce the door-to-balloon time. A **seamless transition** from the emergency department to the catheterization lab is essential.
- **Key Considerations**:
    - **Antithrombotic Therapy**: Early administration of **aspirin** and **P2Y12 inhibitors** (e.g., **clopidogrel**, **ticagrelor**) is essential. If fibrinolysis is used, adjunctive **anticoagulation** (e.g., **enoxaparin**) should be considered.
    - **Anticoagulation**: Use **heparin** or **bivalirudin** during PCI for optimal results.

Life-Threatening Arrhythmias

*Life-threatening arrhythmias, such as **ventricular fibrillation (VF)** and **ventricular tachycardia (VT)**, are major causes of cardiac arrest. Early recognition and treatment are crucial for survival.*

- **Ventricular Fibrillation (VF):**
    - **Pearl**: VF is often the result of **ischemic heart disease** and can lead to sudden cardiac arrest. The absence of a palpable pulse and unresponsiveness are key signs.
    - **Management**: Immediate **defibrillation** (via **AED** or **manual defibrillator**) is the first-line therapy. Early CPR (cardiopulmonary resuscitation) should be initiated if defibrillation is not immediately available.
    - After stabilization, consider **antiarrhythmic drugs** (e.g., **amiodarone**, **lidocaine**) to prevent recurrent VF.
- **Ventricular Tachycardia (VT):**
    - **Pearl**: Monomorphic VT with a **pulse** can be managed with **antiarrhythmic drugs** (e.g., **amiodarone**, **procainamide**). If the patient is unstable, **synchronized cardioversion** is required.
    - **Management: Polymorphic VT** (e.g., **torsades de pointes**) may require **magnesium sulfate** along with **antiarrhythmic therapy**.
- **Bradyarrhythmias:**
    - **Pearl: Symptomatic bradycardia** (e.g., due to **sinus node dysfunction** or **AV block**) may require **atropine** and/or **temporary pacing** (via transcutaneous or transvenous pacing).

- **Management**: If atropine is ineffective, consider **temporary pacing** or in severe cases, permanent pacemaker placement.

CHAPTER 14: SPECIAL POPULATIONS IN CARDIOLOGY

Cardiovascular diseases present unique challenges in different patient populations due to varying physiological conditions, risk factors, and management strategies.

Cardiovascular Diseases In Pregnancy

Pregnancy induces significant physiological changes that can affect cardiovascular function.

Pregnant women are at an increased risk for certain cardiovascular conditions, including **hypertension, pre-eclampsia, peripartum cardiomyopathy**, and **arrhythmias**.

- **Cardiac Physiology During Pregnancy**:
    - **Pearl**: Pregnancy results in increased **cardiac output** (up to 50% higher) and **plasma volume** (up to 40% higher), with decreased systemic vascular resistance due to hormonal changes. These changes place additional strain on the heart, particularly in women with pre-existing heart conditions.
    - **Key Consideration**: Monitoring **blood pressure, heart rate**, and **fluid status** is essential during prenatal visits to detect early signs of cardiac distress.
- **Hypertensive Disorders**:
    - **Pearl**: Hypertension in pregnancy, including

gestational **hypertension** and **pre-eclampsia**, can increase the risk of maternal and fetal complications, such as **stroke**, **eclampsia**, and **fetal growth restriction**.
- **Management:** Blood pressure control is key. **Methyldopa, labetalol,** and **nifedipine** are often considered safe for use during pregnancy. **ACE inhibitors** and **ARBs** should be avoided.

- **Peripartum Cardiomyopathy:**
  - **Pearl:** This rare condition typically occurs in the last month of pregnancy or within 5 months postpartum, presenting with heart failure and a reduced ejection fraction.
  - **Management: Diuretics, ACE inhibitors,** and **beta-blockers** may be used cautiously, and **anticoagulation** may be indicated if there is associated **left ventricular thrombus**. Prompt cardiology consultation is crucial.

- **Arrhythmias in Pregnancy:**
  - **Pearl: Atrial fibrillation** and **supraventricular tachycardia** (SVT) are more common in pregnancy, often due to increased adrenergic activity.
  - **Management:** The first-line treatment is **vagal maneuvers**. If pharmacologic treatment is required, **beta-blockers** (e.g., **metoprolol**) are considered safe. **Digoxin** and **amiodarone** should be used cautiously and only when absolutely necessary.

- **Postpartum Considerations:**
  - **Pearl:** Close monitoring is required after delivery, particularly in women with a history of **pre-eclampsia**, **hypertension**, or

cardiomyopathy, as these conditions may evolve or worsen in the postpartum period.

Cardiology Considerations In The Elderly

*The elderly population is at high risk for developing cardiovascular diseases, including **hypertension**, **heart failure**, **atrial fibrillation**, and **coronary artery disease**.*

Aging-related physiological changes can complicate diagnosis and management.

- **Age-related Cardiac Changes**:
    - **Pearl**: Aging results in **stiffening** of the heart and vasculature, leading to **increased systolic blood pressure**, **reduced diastolic filling**, and decreased myocardial reserve. These changes can exacerbate heart failure symptoms and contribute to **isolated systolic hypertension**.
    - **Management**: Regular monitoring of **blood pressure**, **lipid profile**, and **electrocardiogram (ECG)** is crucial to detect early signs of cardiac disease in elderly patients.
- **Heart Failure in the Elderly**:
    - **Pearl**: Both **heart failure with reduced ejection fraction (HFrEF)** and **heart failure with preserved ejection fraction (HFpEF)** are common in the elderly. HFpEF is particularly prevalent due to **diastolic dysfunction** and increased left ventricular stiffness.
    - **Management**: The cornerstone of treatment for HFrEF includes **ACE inhibitors, beta-blockers**, and **diuretics**. For HFpEF, management focuses on controlling **blood pressure**, **diabetes**, and **atrial fibrillation**.
- **Atrial Fibrillation**:

- **Pearl**: **Atrial fibrillation (AF)** is highly prevalent in the elderly, often leading to increased risk of **stroke** and **heart failure**.
- **Management**: **Rate control** (e.g., **beta-blockers, calcium channel blockers**) is preferred for stable patients. **Anticoagulation** (e.g., **warfarin, dabigatran**) should be based on the **CHA2DS2-VASc** score to prevent thromboembolic events.

- **Polypharmacy Considerations**:
  - **Pearl**: Elderly patients are often on multiple medications, increasing the risk of **drug interactions, adverse effects**, and **non-adherence**. **Careful medication reconciliation** is important.
  - **Management**: Review medications regularly, including diuretics, antihypertensives, antiarrhythmic drugs, and anticoagulants. Adjust dosages as necessary, especially in those with impaired renal function.

- **Frailty and Cardiac Surgery**:
  - **Pearl**: Frailty is associated with worse outcomes after cardiac surgery in the elderly. Preoperative assessment should include an evaluation of physical function and nutritional status.
  - **Management**: Consider **minimally invasive** techniques when possible, and optimize medical management to reduce the need for surgery in high-risk patients.

Sports Cardiology: Pre-Participation Screening

CARDIOLOGY PEARLS

Cardiovascular evaluation is essential for athletes to ensure their safety during physical activities and competitive sports.

Early detection of cardiac abnormalities can help prevent sudden cardiac death (SCD) and other complications.

- **Pre-participation Screening**:
    - **Pearl**: A detailed **history** and **physical examination** are the first steps in screening athletes. Family history of sudden cardiac death or inherited cardiac conditions (e.g., **hypertrophic cardiomyopathy, arrhythmogenic right ventricular cardiomyopathy**) is particularly important.
    - **Key Screening Elements**:
        - **History**: Ask about episodes of **syncope, dizziness**, or **chest pain** during exercise.
        - **Physical Exam**: Look for signs of **hypertrophic cardiomyopathy** (e.g., **systolic murmur**), **arrhythmias**, or **Marfan syndrome** (e.g., **tall stature, long fingers**).
- **Electrocardiogram (ECG)**:
    - **Pearl**: An **ECG** should be performed as part of routine screening for athletes, especially those involved in high-intensity or contact sports. However, normal athletes may have **benign ECG findings** like **early repolarization** or **sinus arrhythmia**, which should not be mistaken for pathology.
    - **Management**: A **negative ECG** does not rule out conditions like **arrhythmogenic right**

ventricular cardiomyopathy (ARVC) or **long QT syndrome**, so additional testing may be required based on clinical suspicion.

- **Echocardiogram:**
    - **Pearl**: An **echocardiogram** may be necessary for athletes with abnormal findings on history, physical exam, or ECG. This is particularly important for detecting **hypertrophic cardiomyopathy**, **aortic aneurysm**, and **valvular abnormalities**.
    - **Management**: **Hypertrophic cardiomyopathy** requires restriction from competitive sports, while **aortic aneurysm** or **dilated cardiomyopathy** may require further assessment to determine risk of sudden cardiac death (SCD).
- **Exercise Testing:**
    - **Pearl**: **Exercise testing** can assess exercise tolerance and uncover arrhythmias or ischemia that may not be evident at rest.
    - **Management**: **Stress echocardiography** or **cardiac MRI** may be useful in athletes with a history of unexplained exertional syncope or chest pain.
- **When to Restrict Participation:**
    - **Pearl**: Athletes with a history of **syncope**, **chest pain**, or **family history of sudden cardiac death** should be evaluated more thoroughly before being cleared for sports. Any athlete with a diagnosed **cardiomyopathy, arrhythmia**, or **significant valvular heart disease** should be restricted from competitive sports.
    - **Management**: Recommendations vary based

on the condition. For example, athletes with **hypertrophic cardiomyopathy** should be restricted from high-intensity and contact sports due to an increased risk of SCD.

ABOUT THE AUTHOR

Dr Essam Abdelhakim

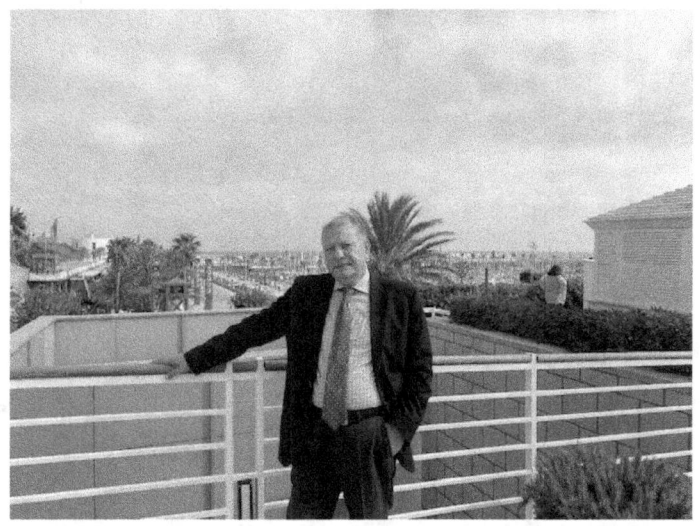

Senior Consultant and Expert in Medical Education

www.ingramcontent.com/pod-product-compliance
Lightning Source LLC
Chambersburg PA
CBHW071105240526
45469CB00006BD/2331